HERBAL REMEDIES

FOR

I0408970

DOG HEALTH

OVER 35 NATURAL HEALINGS FOR CANINE COMPANIONS

BY

CARLOS PHIL

CONTENTS

CHAPTER 1

INTRODUCTION

Welcome to "Herbal Remedies for Dog Health." In this guide, we'll treat comprehensively the world of natural solutions to enhance the well-being of your furry companions. As the owner and lover of pets, we understand the deep love we share with our dogs and the desire to provide them with the best possible care. Herbal treatments offer a holistic approach to addressing various health concerns, promoting vitality, and supporting their overall quality of life.

Throughout this book, we will explore a wide range of natural healings that can help in playing a significant role in maintaining your dog's health.

From soothing digestive issues and nurturing skin irritations to easing joint discomfort and alleviating stress, these natural home-made remedies have the potential to become valuable tools in your pet care arsenal.

Before we delve into this herbal journey, it's crucial to emphasize the importance of safety. While herbs can offer numerous benefits, not all remedies are suitable for every dog, and proper dosages must be considered. Always consult with your veterinarian before introducing any new herbs or treatments, especially if your dog has pre-existing health conditions or is taking medication.

In the modern world, as the interest in natural and holistic approaches to healthcare continues to improve, many pet owners are seeking alternatives to traditional treatments for their canine companions. Herbal remedies have been used for centuries by different cultures to address a wide array of health problems, and now, these time-tested solutions are finding their way into our pets' lives.

Our dogs are more than just pets; they are beloved members of our families. We share our lives, homes, and hearts with them, and their well-being is of great importance. As responsible dog owners, we strive to provide them with the proper care possible, and that includes exploring all available options for maintaining their health.

The journey of using herbal remedies for your dog's health is not just about finding quick fixes or magical cures. It's about understanding the natural world and its potential to complement conventional veterinary care. While modern medicine certainly has its place, herbal remedies offer an alternative path that focuses on prevention, balance, and wellness.

Throughout the pages of this manual, we will not only introduce you to specific herbs that can benefit your dog's health, but we will also delve into the art of creating herbal preparations. From herbal teas and tinctures to soothing balms and nourishing treats, you'll learn how to harness the power of nature in ways that are safe and effective.

However, it's important to note that this book is not a replacement for professional veterinary advice. Herbal remedies should always be used in addition with the guidance of a qualified veterinarian who understands your dog's unique health requirements.

So, whether you're seeking to address a specific health concern or simply want to improve your dog's overall vitality, **"Herbal Remedies for Dog Health"** will serve as your guide on this journey of exploration. As you turn the pages, may you find inspiration, knowledge, and a deeper connection with the natural world, all aimed at enriching the lives of your beloved four-legged friends. By gaining insights into the world of herbal remedies for dogs and combining this knowledge with professional veterinary guidance, you'll be empowered to make right decisions about your dog's well-being. Let's focus on this enlightening exploration of herbal remedies and unlock the secrets to improving your dog's health naturally.

CHAPTER 2

COMMON HERBS FOR DOG HEALTH

Dogs, like humans, can benefit from the incredible healing properties of different herbs. In this chapter, we'll delve into the world of common herbs that can play a pivotal role in supporting your dog's well-being. From promoting digestive health to soothing skin irritations and assist in providing relief from joint discomfort, these herbs are nature's gifts that can improve your dog's quality of life.

Benefits of Herbal Remedies

Before we explore individual herbs, it's essential to know why herbal remedies are gaining popularity among pet owners. Herbal solutions offer a holistic approach to dog health, treating not just the symptoms but also the underlying causes of various illness. These remedies work in harmony with your dog's body, often providing a gentler and more natural alternative to traditional treatments.

Precautions and Dosage

While herbs can offer numerous benefits, it's use to use them with care and moderation. Not all herbs are safe for dogs, and wrong dosages can lead to adverse effects. Consulting with a veterinarian experienced in herbal medicine is paramount to ensure the safety and efficacy of any remedies you choose to administer to your dog. This section will provide you with essential information to ensure that you're using herbs correctly and responsibly.

Now, let's explore some of the most common and versatile herbs that can improve your dog's overall health and well-being:

Peppermint for Upset Stomach

Peppermint is popular for its soothing properties and its capacity to calm digestive discomfort in dogs. Whether it's a case of indigestion, gas, or mild stomach upset, peppermint can give relief and promote healthy digestion.

Chamomile for Digestive Calm

Chamomile is a gentle herb that works wonders for dogs with digestive issues. Its anti-inflammatory and calming properties can help palliate stomach cramps, nausea, and even anxiety-related digestive disturbances.

Throughout this chapter, we'll keep to explore a variety of herbs, their benefits, and how they can be used to support your dog's health naturally. Remember, each dog is unique, and what works well for one may not work for another. By arming yourself with knowledge about these common herbs, you'll be better equipped to make right decisions about your dog's well-being.

CHAPTER 3

HERBS FOR DIGESTIVE HEALTH

A healthy digestive system is fundamental to your dog's overall well-being. Just like in humans, the digestive tract plays an important role in absorbing nutrients, excreting waste, and maintaining a strong immune system. In this chapter, we will explore a selection of herbs that can offer support for various digestive issues your dog may face. From upset stomachs to indigestion, these natural remedies can provide relief and contribute to a balanced digestive system.

Peppermint for Upset Stomach

Scientific Name: Mentha Piperita

Benefits: Peppermint is known for its ability to ease stomach discomfort, eliminate bloating, and alleviate gas. It contains compounds that relax the muscles of the gastrointestinal tract, helping to relieve spasms and cramps.

Usage: Peppermint can be administered as a mild infusion or mixed into dog-friendly treats. It's important to use only moderate amounts, as excessive peppermint can lead to digestive upset.

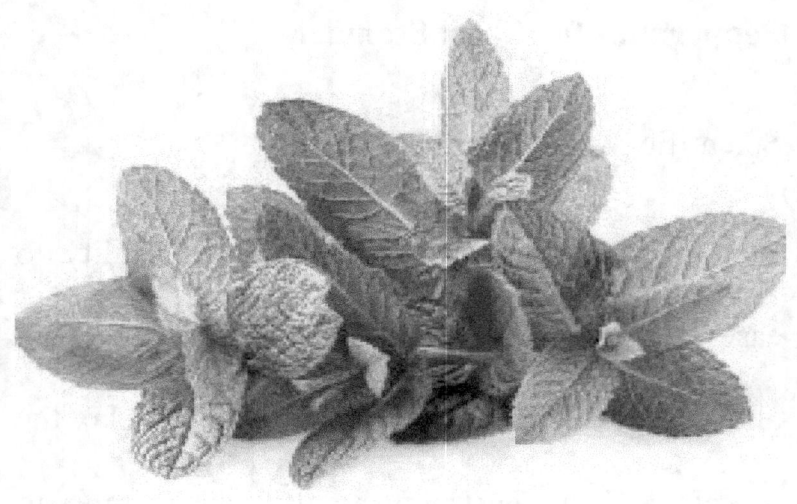

Chamomile for Digestive Calm

Scientific Name: Matricaria Chamomilla

Benefits: Chamomile is a gentle herb with anti-inflammatory properties that can soothe an upset stomach and lower gastrointestinal irritation. It also has calming effects that can help with stress-related digestive problems.

Usage: Chamomile tea can be prepared and cooled before offering it to your dog. Additionally, chamomile extracts can be found in certain dog digestive supplements.

By exploring these herbs for digestive health, keep in mind that individual dogs may react differently. It's recommended to begin with small doses and monitor your dog's response. If your dog has a history of gastrointestinal issues or is on medication, consult with a veterinarian before introducing any herbal remedies. The goal is to provide your dog with a comfortable and well-functioning digestive system, improving their overall quality of life.

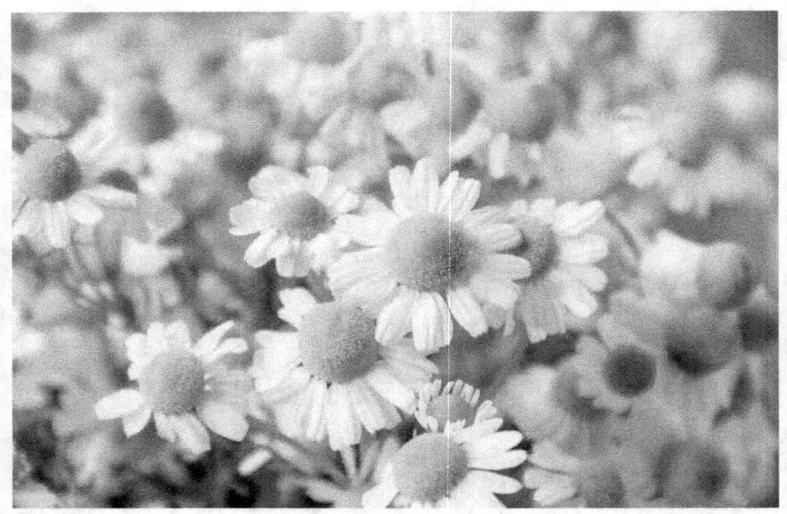

Ginger for Nausea and Bloating

Scientific Name: Zingiber Officinale

Benefits: Ginger is well-known for its anti-nausea properties and its capacity to palliate bloating. It can help calm an upset stomach and reduce feelings of nausea, making it particularly useful during car rides or for dogs prone to motion sickness.

Usage: Fresh ginger can be grated and added in small amounts to your dog's food. Alternatively, ginger tea can be made and administered in moderation.

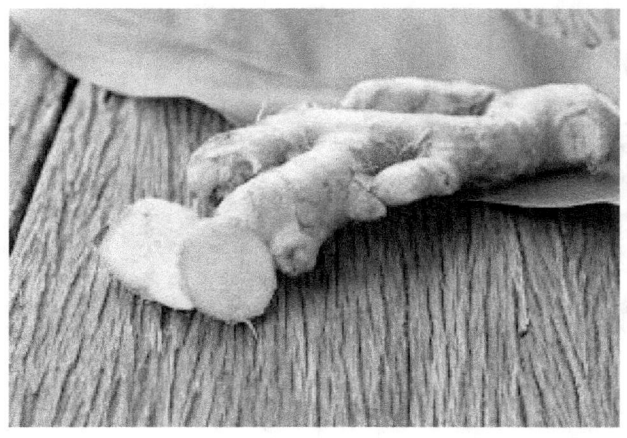

Fennel for Digestive Support

Scientific Name: Foeniculum Vulgare

Benefits: Fennel is often used to aid digestion, reduce gas, and palliate indigestion. It can help soothe the digestive tract and promote healthy bowel movements.

Usage: Fennel seeds can be ground and added to your dog's meals. Fennel tea can also be prepared by steeping the seeds in warm water.

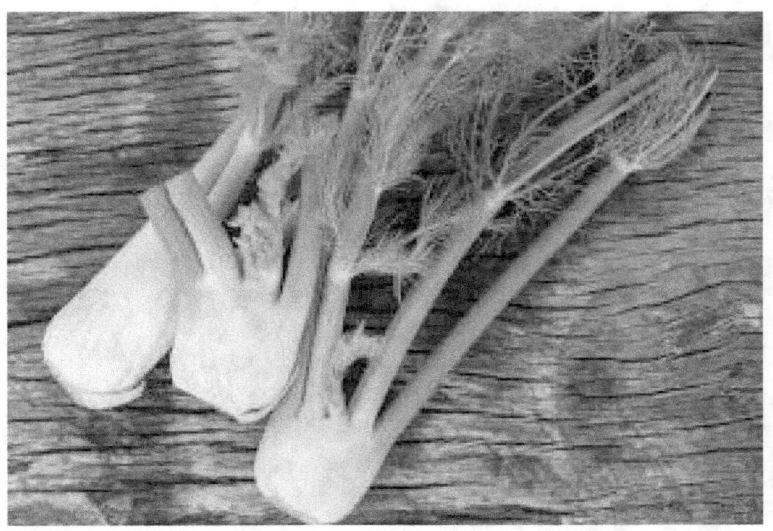

Dandelion for Liver Health

Scientific Name: Taraxacum Officinale

Benefits: Dandelion is a natural diuretic that can in supporting the liver and promote healthy bile production. It's beneficial for dogs with liver disorders or those in need of detoxification.

23

Usage: Dandelion leaves can be added to your dog's diet in small amounts. Dandelion root can be dried, crushed, and sprinkled over meals.

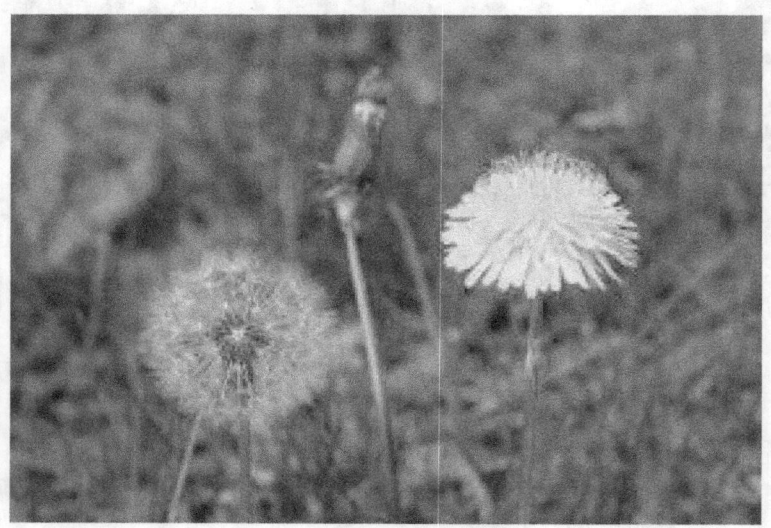

Slippery Elm for Digestive Soothing

Scientific Name: Ulmus Rubra

Benefits: Slippery elm is known for its soothing properties on the digestive tract. It can help to palliate inflammation, irritation, and discomfort.

Usage: Slippery elm powder can be mixed with water to create a gel-like substance that can be added to your dog's food.

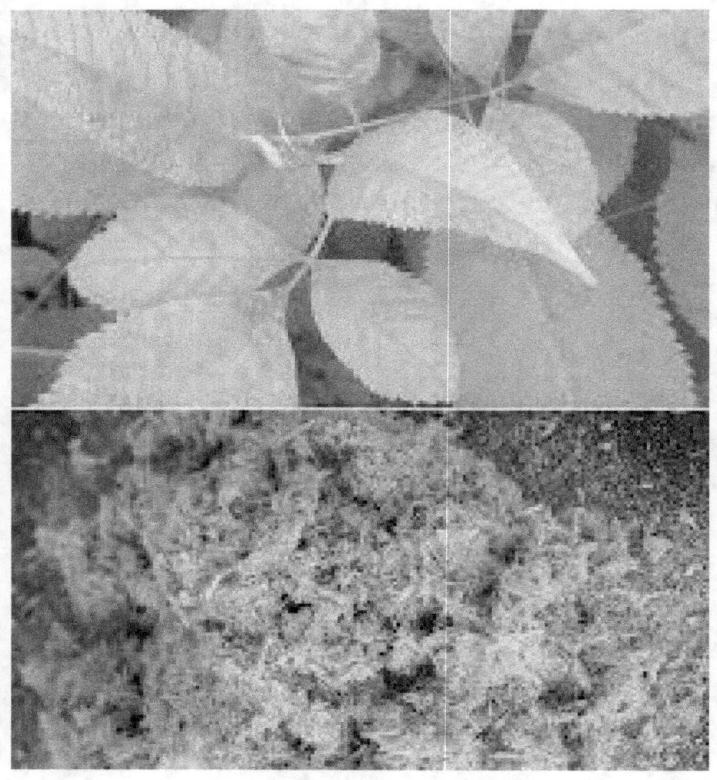

Creating Herbal Blends

Combining these herbs in careful proportions can create effective herbal solutions tailored to your dog's specific needs. However, it's important to consult with a veterinarian or a professional experienced in herbal medicine before creating custom blends. Dosage and compatibility with any existing health conditions or medications need to be taken into account.

Remember, while herbs can put valuable support for digestive health, they are not a substitute for professional veterinary care. If your dog experiences severe or persistent digestive issues, it's crucial to consult with a veterinarian to determine the underlying cause and receive appropriate medication.

As you explore these natural solutions for digestive health, you'll be equipped with valuable knowledge to make informed decisions about your dog's well-being. By incorporating these herbs into your dog's diet with professional assistance, you can add to their comfort, happiness, and overall vitality.

CHAPTER 4

HERBS FOR SKIN AND COAT HEALTH

A lustrous coat and healthy skin are not only signs of a well-cared-for dog but also indicators of their overall vitality. Just like humans, dogs can experience a range of skin issues, from irritations and allergies to dryness and infections. In this chapter, we'll delve into endorsement of herbs that can help promote skin and coat health, addressing common concerns and improving your dog's natural radiance.

Aloe Vera for Skin Irritations

Scientific Name: Aloe Barbadensis Miller

Benefits: Aloe Vera is popular for its soothing and cooling properties. It can provide relief from minor skin irritations, itching, and inflammation. Aloe Vera also contains compounds that support skin healing.

Usage: The gel from a fresh aloe vera leaf can be applied topically to affected areas. Commercial Aloe Vera products should be selected carefully, as some may contain added ingredients that could be harmful to dogs.

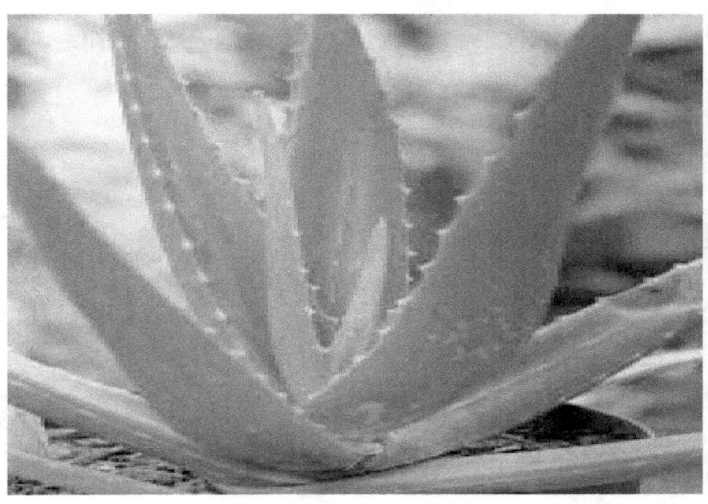

Calendula for Wound Healing

Scientific Name: Calendula Officinalis

Benefits: Calendula possesses anti-inflammatory and antimicrobial properties, making it an excellent herb for promoting wound healing. It can soothe and protect the skin while supporting the regeneration of healthy tissue.

Usage: Calendula oil or salve can be applied topically to minor cuts, scrapes, and irritations. It's important to ensure that the product used is safe for dogs.

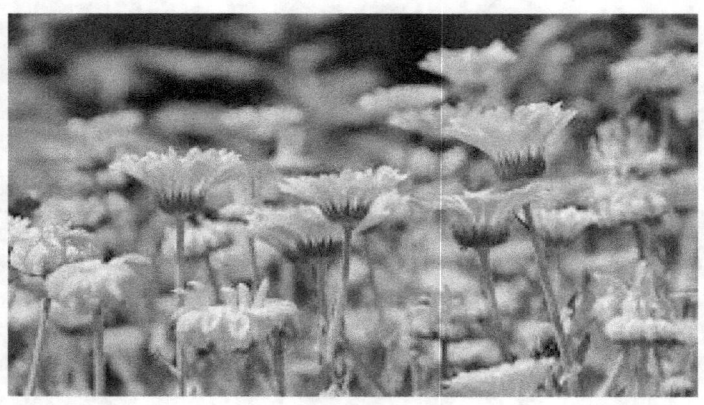

Lavender for Skin Comfort

Scientific Name: Lavandula Angustifolia

Benefits: Lavender is renowned for its calming and antiseptic properties. It can help soothe irritated skin, reduce itching, and provide relief from discomfort caused by minor skin issues.

Usage: Lavender essential oil can be diluted and applied sparingly to the affected area. Alternatively, lavender-infused baths can help provide overall skin comfort.

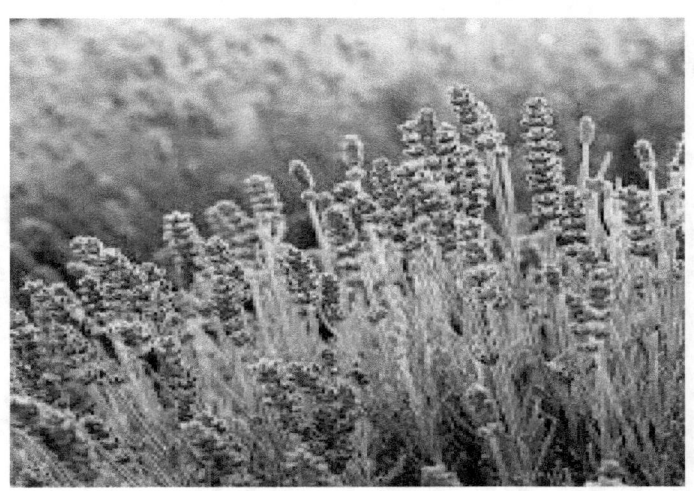

Burdock Root for Skin Health

Scientific Name: Arctium Lappa

Benefits: Burdock root is beneficial for promoting healthy skin from within. It supports detoxification and can help address skin issues caused by impurities in the body.

Usage: Burdock root can be added to your dog's diet in powdered form. It's important to follow prescribed dosages and consult with a veterinarian.

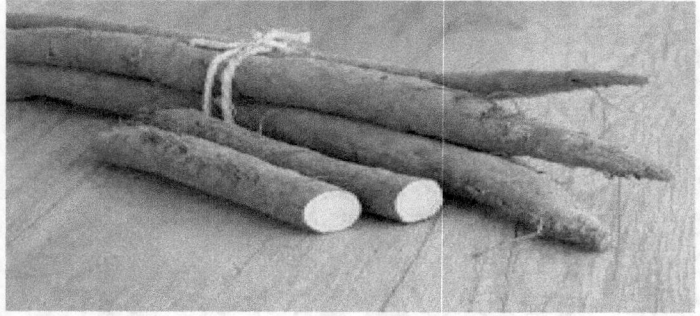

Coconut Oil for Moisturizing

Scientific Name: Cocos Nucifera

Benefits: Coconut oil is a natural moisturizer that can help fight dry and flaky skin. It contains fatty acids that nourish the skin and contribute to a healthy, shiny coat.

Usage: A small amount of coconut oil can be added to your dog's food for internal benefits or applied topically to dry areas.

As you explore these herbs for skin and coat health, remember that individual dogs may react differently. If your dog has a history of skin issues or allergies, consulting with a veterinarian experienced in herbal medicine is recommended.

By incorporating these natural remedies into your dog's care routine, you can contribute to their comfort, confidence, and overall well-being.

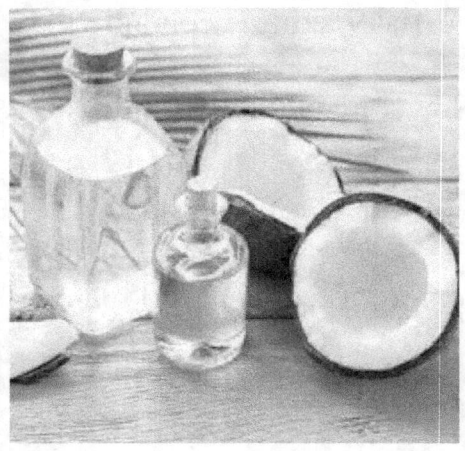

Chamomile for Itch Relief

Scientific Name: Matricaria Chamomilla

Benefits: Chamomile's anti-inflammatory and soothing properties add to skin health as well. It can provide relief from itching and irritation caused by allergies, insect bites, or minor skin rashes.

Usage: Chamomile tea can be brewed, cooled, and applied as a gentle rinse to the affected area. Alternatively, chamomile-infused oils or balms can be used topically.

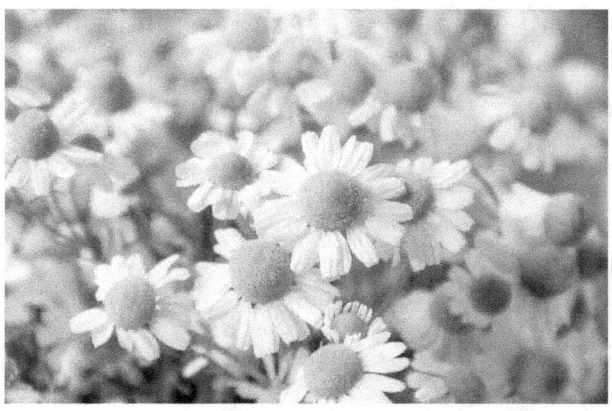

Neem for Skin Protection

Scientific Name: Azadirachta Indica

Benefits: Neem is a powerful herb with natural antibacterial and antifungal properties. It can help protect the skin from infections and support healing of minor wounds or irritations.

Usage: Neem oil can be diluted and applied topically. It's important to use neem in moderation, as its potent properties can be too much for some dogs.

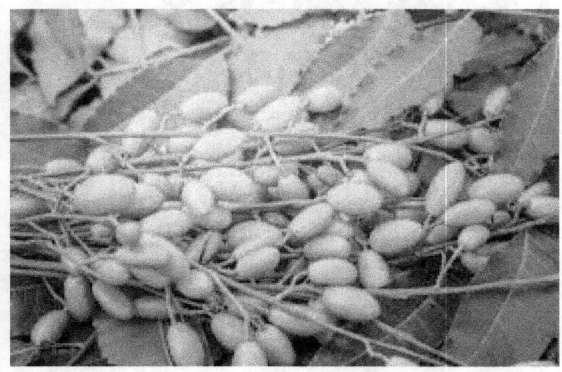

Marshmallow Root for Soothing

Scientific Name: Althaea Officinalis

Benefits: Marshmallow root contains mucilage, a gel-like substance that can provide a soothing and protective layer to irritated skin. It helps palliate itching and discomfort.

Usage: Marshmallow root can be used to create a soothing poultice or added to homemade balms and salves.

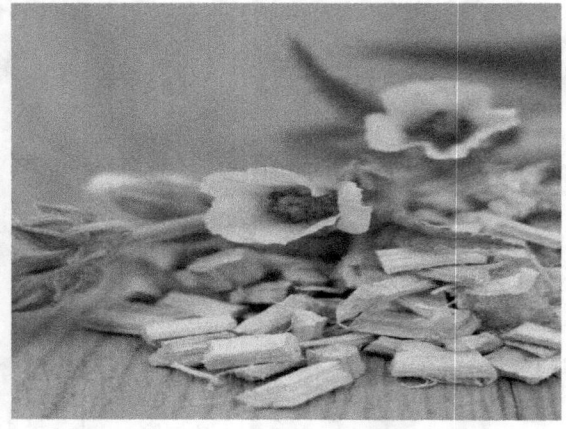

Oatmeal for Soothing Baths

Scientific Name: Avena Sativa

Benefits: Oatmeal is a classic remedy for soothing irritated skin. It can provide relief from itching, inflammation, and dryness, making it ideal for dogs with sensitive skin.

Usage: Finely ground oatmeal can be added to bathwater to create a calming and soothing soak for your dog. After the bath, make sure to rinse thoroughly.

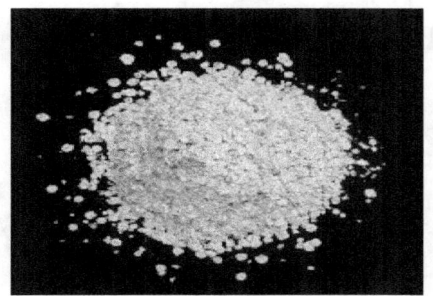

Creating Herbal Infusions

Harnessing the benefits of these herbs for skin and coat health often involves creating herbal infusions or topical applications. Keep in mind that individual dogs may have different sensitivities and reactions. Performing a patch test before applying any new herbal remedy is recommended,

41

especially if your dog has a history of allergies or sensitivities.

Additionally, while herbal remedies can be highly effective, they are not a replacement for professional veterinary care. If your dog experiences severe or persistent skin issues, it's important to consult with a veterinarian to identify the underlying cause and receive appropriate medications.

By incorporating these natural remedies into your dog's care routine, you're not only addressing specific skin and coat concerns but also nurturing their overall well-being. As you embark on this journey of using herbs for skin and coat health, may your dog's comfort and radiance be a testament to the power of nature's remedies.

CHAPTER 5

HERBS FOR JOINT AND MOBILITY SUPPORT

As our beloved canine companions age, maintaining their joint health becomes steadily important. Just like humans, dogs can experience joint discomfort, stiffness, and reduced mobility. In this chapter, we'll explore a selection of herbs that can provide support for your dog's joint health, helping them move comfortably and enjoy an active lifestyle.

Turmeric for Inflammation

Scientific Name: Curcuma Longa

Benefits: Turmeric contains curcumin, a compound with potent anti-inflammatory properties. It can help reduce inflammation in the joints and alleviate discomfort associated with arthritis.

Usage: Turmeric can be added to your dog's food in powdered form or as a supplement. It's often recommended to combine turmeric with black pepper to ease its absorption.

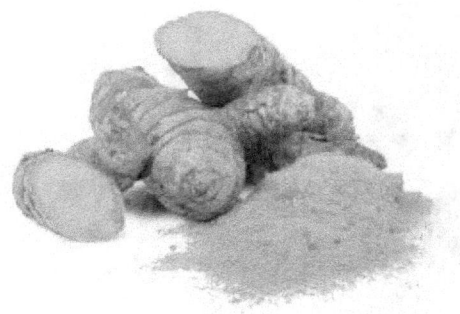

Yucca for Joint Pain

Scientific Name: Yucca Schidigera

Benefits: Yucca contains saponins, compounds that have been shown to have anti-inflammatory effects. It can help reduce joint pain and promote better mobility.

Usage: Yucca supplements are available in various forms, including capsules and liquid extracts. Consult with a veterinarian for proper dosage.

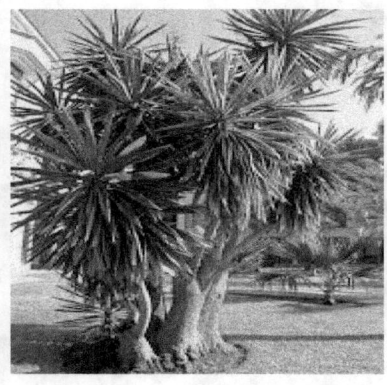

Boswellia for Joint Function

Scientific Name: Boswellia Serrata

Benefits: Boswellia, also known as frankincense, has active compounds that can support joint function and ease stiffness. It's particularly beneficial for dogs with degenerative joint conditions.

Usage: Boswellia supplements are available and can be administered as directed. It's important to choose high-quality products.

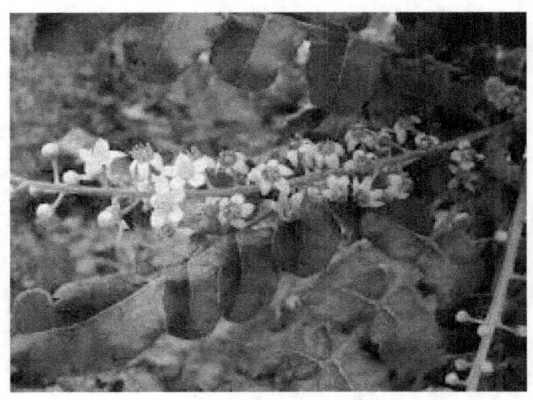

Nettle for Joint Comfort

Scientific Name: Urtica dioica

Benefits: Nettle is rich in nutrients that can support joint health. It contains vitamins, minerals, and antioxidants that help alleviate inflammation and improve overall joint comfort.

Usage: Nettle can be given to dogs in dried or powdered form. It's often included in blends for joint support.

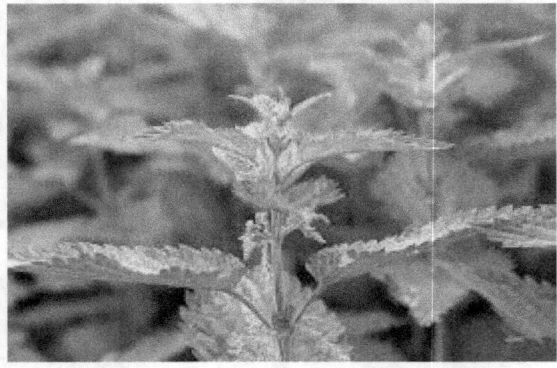

Creating Herbal Blends

Combining these herbs in appropriate proportions can create effective herbal blends tailored to your dog's joint health needs. However, it's important to consult with a veterinarian or herbalist experienced in pet health before creating custom blends. Each dog is unique, and factors such as age, weight, and existing health conditions should be considered.

Remember, while herbs can offer valuable support for joint health, they are not a substitute for professional veterinary care. If your dog is experiencing significant joint issues, it's essential to consult with a veterinarian for a proper diagnosis and treatment plan.

49

By incorporating these natural remedies into your dog's daily routine under the guidance of a professional, you're contributing to their comfort, mobility, and overall well-being.

Devil's Claw for Mobility

Scientific Name: Harpagophytum Procumbens

Benefits: Devil's claw is known for its anti-inflammatory properties and its potential to alleviate joint pain and discomfort. It can help improve mobility and enhance your dog's quality of life.

Usage: Devil's claw supplements are available in various forms, including capsules and powders.

Consulting with a veterinarian is recommended to determine the appropriate dosage.

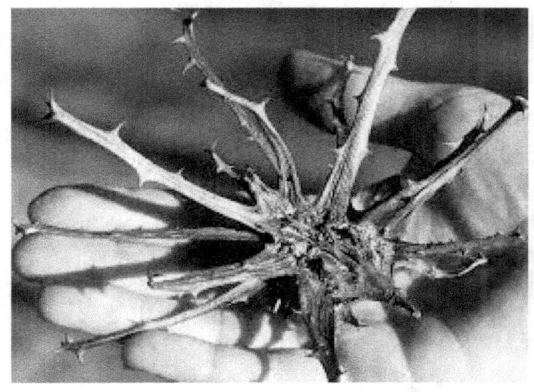

Meadowsweet for Joint Support

Scientific Name: Filipendula Ulmaria

Benefits: Meadowsweet has natural salicylates, which can act as mild pain relievers and provide joint support. It's a gentle option for dogs experiencing mild to moderate discomfort.

51

Usage: Meadowsweet can be made as a tea and added to your dog's water or food. Commercial meadowsweet products should be chosen with care.

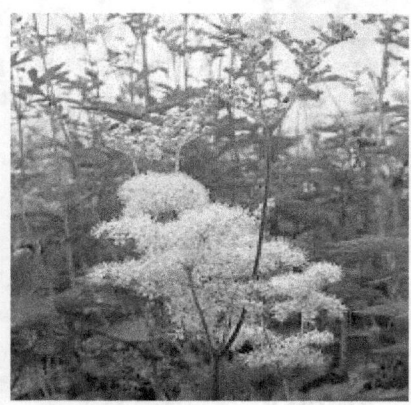

Horsetail for Connective Tissue

Scientific Name: Equisetum Arvense

Benefits: Horsetail is rich in silica, a mineral that supports the health of connective tissues, including joints. It can help manage the integrity of cartilage and promote joint flexibility.

Usage: Horsetail can be given as a supplement in appropriate dosages. It's important to consult with a veterinarian to ensure proper administration.

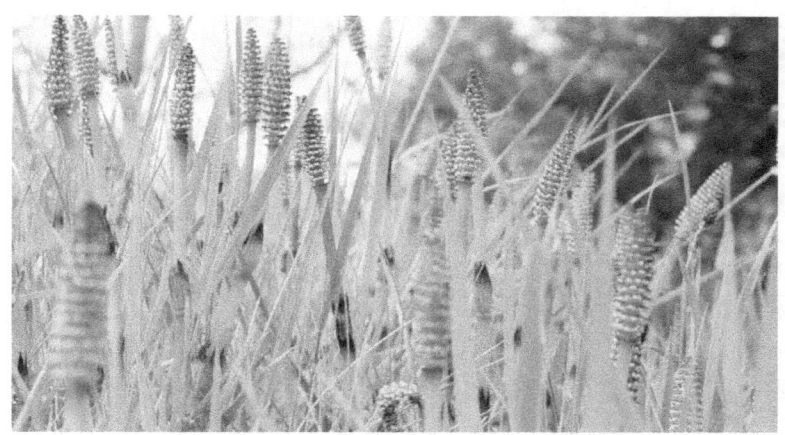

Cayenne for Circulation

Scientific Name: Capsicum annuum

Benefits: Cayenne contains capsaicin, a compound that can improve circulation and provide a warming sensation. Improved circulation can aid in delivering nutrients to the joints and reducing stiffness.

Usage: Cayenne can be incorporated into homemade balms or liniments for topical application. It's essential to use caution and avoid contact with the eyes.

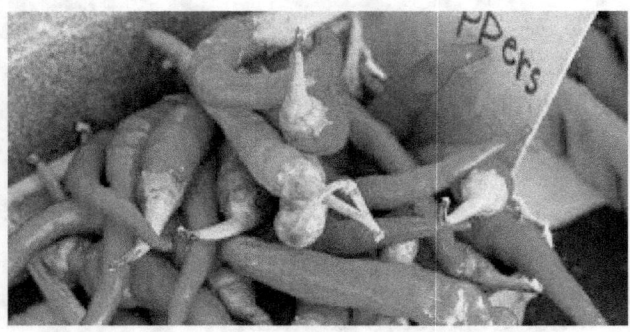

Integrating Herbal Remedies
When considering herbal remedies for joint and mobility support, it's crucial to integrate them into your dog's routine gradually and with professional guidance. Consulting with a veterinarian

experienced in herbal medicine ensures that you're using appropriate herbs and dosages for your dog's specific needs.

Additionally, while herbs can offer valuable assistance, they are most effective when used alongside a holistic approach to joint care. This may include maintaining a healthy weight, providing regular exercise, and ensuring your dog's living environment is comfortable and safe.

As you explore these natural remedies for joint and mobility support, you're taking proactive steps to enhance your dog's comfort and well-being. By fostering healthy joints and promoting mobility, you're enabling your beloved companion to enjoy an active and fulfilling life, even as they age gracefully.

CHAPTER 6

HERBS FOR ANXIETY AND STRESS RELIEF

Dogs, like humans, can experience anxiety and stress due to various factors, such as separation, loud noises, or changes in their environment. In this chapter, we'll treat comprehensively the selection of herbs that can provide natural relief for your dog's anxiety and stress, promoting a sense of calm and well-being.

Valerian Root for Calming

Scientific Name: Valeriana Officinalis

Benefits: Valerian root is renowned for its calming effects on the nervous system. It can help reduce anxiety, soothe restlessness, and promote relaxation in dogs.

Usage: Valerian root supplements are available in various forms, including capsules and tinctures. Consulting with a veterinarian is recommended to determine the appropriate dosage.

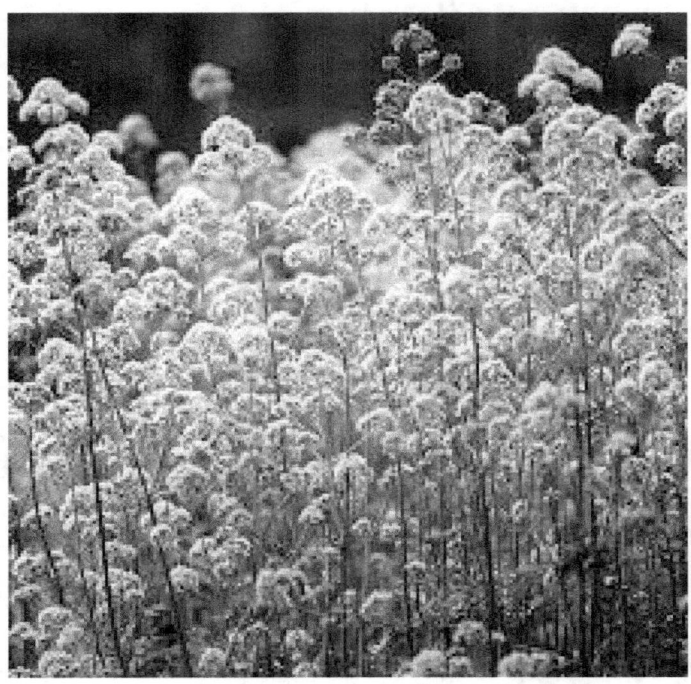

Chamomile for Relaxation

Scientific Name: Matricaria chamomilla

Benefits: Chamomile's gentle properties extend to anxiety relief as well. It can help calm nervous tension, reduce irritability, and support relaxation in dogs.

Usage: Chamomile tea can be made and given to your dog. Additionally, chamomile extracts can be found in certain dog supplements.

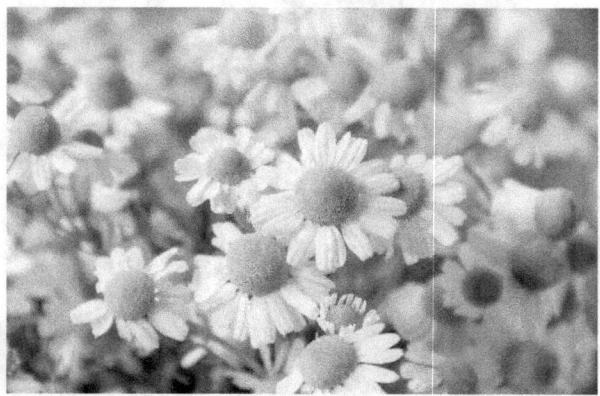

Lavender for Tranquility

Scientific Name: Lavandula angustifolia

Benefits: Lavender is well-known for its soothing scent and calming effects. It can help palliate stress, anxiety, and restlessness in dogs, promoting a sense of tranquility.

Usage: Lavender essential oil can be diffused in the environment or diluted for topical use. It's important to ensure proper dilution and avoid direct contact with your dog's skin.

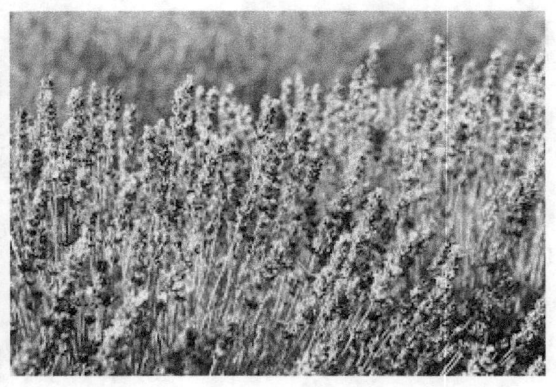

Passionflower for Stress Reduction

Scientific Name: Passiflora Incarnata

Benefits: Passionflower is known for its capacity to reduce stress and anxiety by promoting relaxation. It can help ease nervous tension and provide relief from overactive behavior.

Usage: Passionflower supplements are available in various forms. Consulting with a veterinarian will help determine the appropriate dosage.

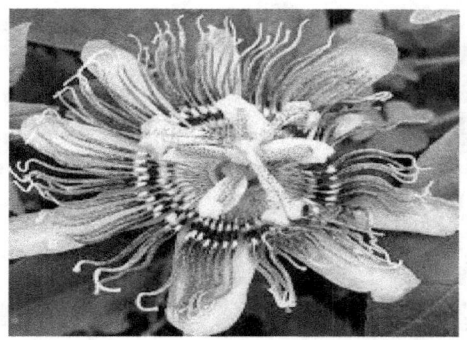

Creating a Calming Environment

In addition to using herbal remedies, creating a calming environment for your dog can further contribute to their well-being. Providing a quiet and safe space, engaging in regular exercise, and maintaining a consistent routine can all help reduce anxiety and stress levels.

Remember, while herbs can offer valuable support, they are not a substitute for professional veterinary advice. If your dog's anxiety is severe or persistent,

63

consulting with a veterinarian is important to manage the underlying causes and develop a comprehensive treatment plan.

By incorporating these natural remedies into your dog's routine, you're promoting emotional balance and helping them navigate the challenges of anxiety and stress with greater ease and comfort.

Lemon Balm for Nervousness

Scientific Name: Melissa Officinalis

Benefits: Lemon balm is known for its calming and mood-balancing abilities. It can help reduce nervousness, restlessness, and promote relaxation in dogs.

Usage: Lemon balm tea can be made and given to your dog. Alternatively, lemon balm extracts can be added to food or water.

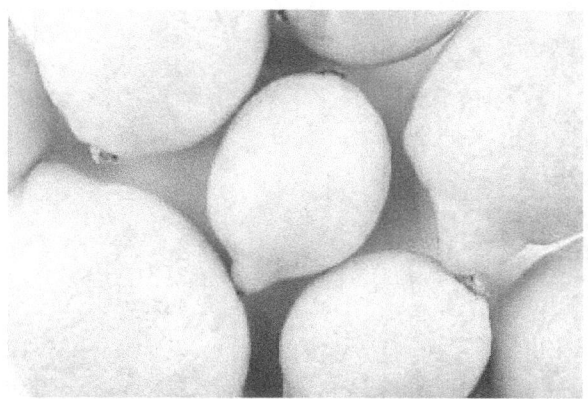

Skullcap for Anxiety

Scientific Name: Scutellaria Lateriflora

Benefits: Skullcap is a gentle herb that can provide relief from anxiety and nervous tension. It can help calm an overactive mind and support emotional well-being.

Usage: Skullcap supplements are available and can be administered as directed. Consulting with a veterinarian is recommended.

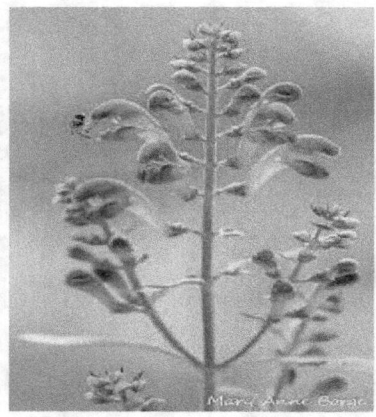

Ashwagandha for Adaptation

Scientific Name: Withania Somnifera

Benefits: Ashwagandha is an adaptogenic herb that can help dogs to cope better with stressors. It enhance the body's ability to adapt and respond to various challenges.

Usage: Ashwagandha supplements can be given to dogs under professional guidance. Dosage recommendations should be followed.

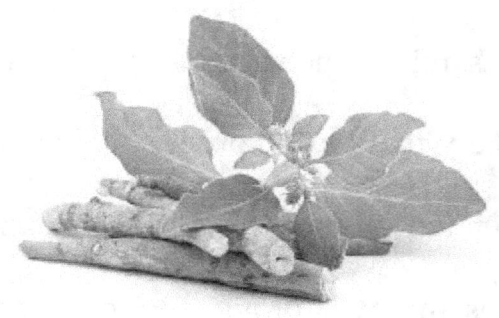

Lavender Aromatherapy

In addition to topical application, lavender aromatherapy can be a valuable tool for anxiety relief. Lavender essential oil can be diffused in the air or applied to a fabric item placed in your dog's sleeping area. The calming scent of lavender can help create a serene atmosphere and promote relaxation.

Creating a Calming Routine

Consistency is key when using herbal remedies for anxiety and stress relief. Incorporate these herbs into your dog's daily routine and observe how they respond. Pay attention to your dog's behavior and body language, as this will provide insights into the effectiveness of the remedies.

While herbs can offer significant benefits, it's important to remember that each dog is unique. Some herbs may be more effective for certain dogs than others. Consulting with a veterinarian or herbalist experienced in pet health can help you tailor a suitable approach to your dog's specific needs.

By incorporating these natural remedies and strategies into your dog's care routine, you're providing them with tools to manage anxiety and stress in a holistic and compassionate way. Your efforts will contribute to a happier, calmer, and more emotionally balanced canine companion.

CHAPTER 7

HERBS FOR IMMUNE SYSTEM BOOST

A robust immune system is essential for your dog's overall health and resilience. Just like humans, dogs can benefit from natural immune-supporting herbs that help fend off infections and maintain their well-being. In this chapter, we'll explore a selection of herbs that can contribute to enhancing your dog's immune system, ensuring they're better equipped to face various health challenges.

Echinacea for Immune Support

Scientific Name: Echinacea Purpurea

Benefits: Echinacea is well-known for its immune-boosting properties. It can help stimulate immune response, support the body's defense mechanisms, and assist in combating infections.

Usage: Echinacea supplements are available in various forms, including capsules and tinctures. Consulting with a veterinarian will help determine the appropriate dosage.

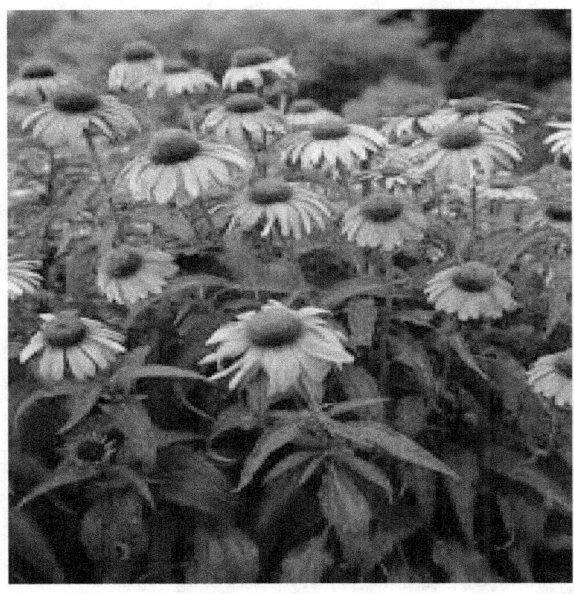

Astragalus for Overall Health

Scientific Name: Astragalus Membranaceus

Benefits: Astragalus is an adaptogenic herb that can improve the immune system's functioning. It supports overall health and vitality, helping dogs better adapt to stressors.

Usage: Astragalus supplements can be administered under professional guidance. Dosage recommendations should be followed.

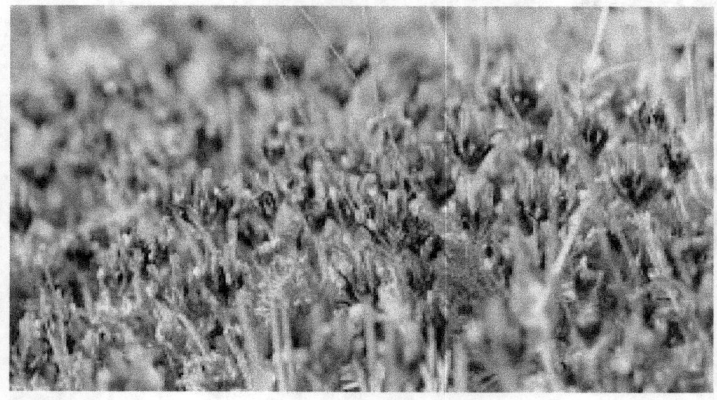

Garlic for Antimicrobial Support

Scientific Name: Allium sativum

Benefits: Garlic has compounds with antimicrobial properties that can help fight off infections. It also supports immune function by promoting white blood cell activity.

Usage: Garlic can be included in small amounts in your dog's diet. It's important to consult with a veterinarian, especially for dogs with certain health conditions.

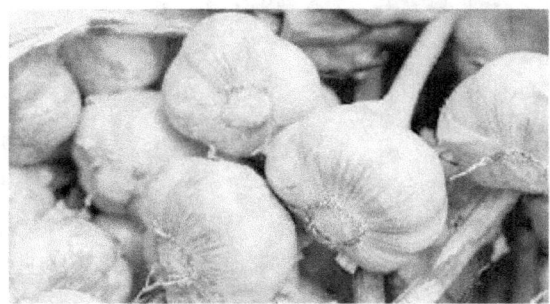

Reishi Mushroom for Immune Modulation

Scientific Name: Ganoderma lucidum

Benefits: Reishi mushroom is an immune-modulating herb that can help balance the immune system's response. It supports overall immune function and vitality.

Usage: Reishi mushroom supplements are available and can be given to dogs under professional guidance.

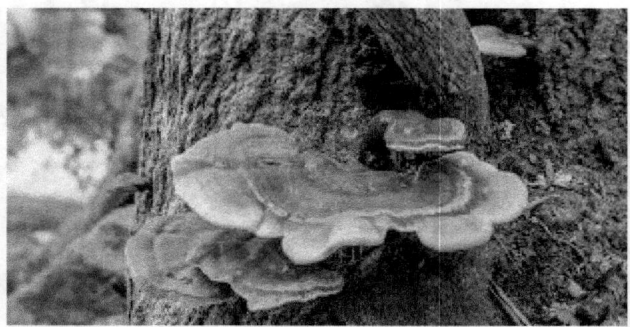

Creating a Balanced Diet

In addition to using immune-supporting herbs, maintaining a balanced and nutritious diet is essential for your dog's immune health. Provide a diet rich in high-quality protein, fresh fruits, and vegetables to supply essential nutrients that support immune function.

Remember, while herbs can offer valuable support, they are not a substitute for professional veterinary care. If your dog has a weakened immune system or underlying health conditions, consulting with a veterinarian is important to determine the best approach to immune support.

By incorporating these natural remedies into your dog's routine, you're helping them maintain a strong and resilient immune system, ensuring they can enjoy optimal health and vitality.

Olive Leaf for Antioxidant Protection

Scientific Name: Olea Europaea

Benefits: Olive leaf is rich in antioxidants that can help guard cells from damage caused by free radicals. It supports immune health by promoting overall cellular well-being.

Usage: Olive leaf supplements can be offered to dogs to provide antioxidant support. Consulting with a veterinarian will help determine appropriate dosages.

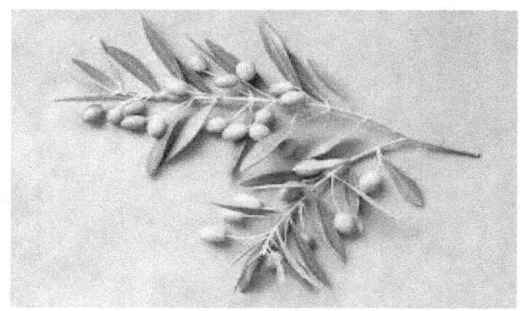

Licorice Root for Immune Modulation

Scientific Name: Glycyrrhiza glabra

Benefits: Licorice root is an adaptogenic herb that can help modulate the immune response. It supports immune balance and overall health.

Usage: Licorice root supplements can be administered under professional guidance. Dosage recommendations should be followed.

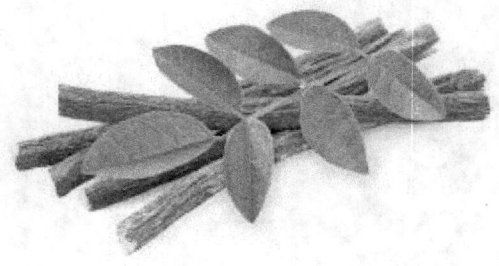

Thyme for Respiratory Health

Scientific Name: Thymus Vulgaris

Benefits: Thyme has compounds that support respiratory health and can help fend off infections. It's particularly beneficial during times of seasonal challenges.

Usage: Thyme can be used to prepare herbal infusions or incorporated into your dog's diet in small amounts.

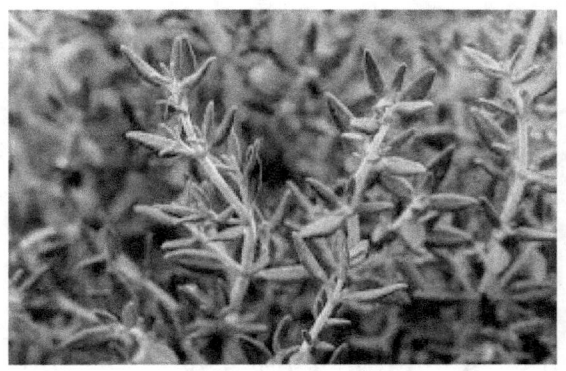

Mushrooms for Immune Enhancement

In addition to reishi mushroom, other mushrooms such as shiitake, maitake, and turkey tail are valued for their immune-boosting properties. These mushrooms have compounds that support immune function and overall vitality.

Usage: Mushroom supplements or blends can be given to dogs under professional guidance.

79

Different mushrooms have varying benefits, so it's important to choose the right ones for your dog's needs.

Holistic Immune Support

Immune health is a multifaceted aspect of your dog's overall well-being. In addition to using immune-supporting herbs, ensuring your dog's environment is clean, providing regular exercise, and minimizing stress all contribute to a strong immune system.

While herbs can offer significant immune support, it's important to consult with a veterinarian to determine the appropriate approach for your dog's individual health needs. A qualified professional can help you create a comprehensive plan that includes herbal remedies and other wellness strategies.

By incorporating these natural remedies and strategies into your dog's care routine, you're taking proactive steps to strengthen their immune system, helping them enjoy a healthier, more vibrant life. Your dedication to their well-being will be reflected in their overall vitality and resilience.

CHAPTER 8

CREATING HERBAL PREPARATIONS

As you delve into the world of herbal solutions for your dog's health, it's important to not only understand the herbs themselves but also how to transform them into effective and safe preparations. In this chapter, we'll explore the art of creating herbal remedies from scratch, empowering you to craft tailored solutions that support your dog's well-being.

Infusions and Teas

Herbal Infusions: Infusions involve steeping herbs in hot water to extract their beneficial compounds. This gentle method is perfect for leaves, flowers, and delicate plant parts. After steeping, strain the infusion and offer it to your dog.

Usage: Herbal infusions can be added to your dog's water, mixed into their food, or applied topically as a soothing rinse.

Decoctions for Rooty Goodness

Herbal Decoctions: For tougher plant parts like roots and bark, decoctions are the way to go. Simmer the herbs in water for an extended period to draw out their therapeutic properties. Strain the liquid and let it cool before use.

Usage: Decoctions can be incorporated into your dog's meals or used in topical applications for specific issues.

Tinctures: Potent Extracts

Herbal Tinctures: Tinctures are concentrated extracts made by soaking herbs in alcohol or glycerin. They're powerful and convenient, making it easy to administer herbs to your dog.

Usage: Tinctures can be added to food, water, or directly into your dog's mouth. Follow dosage guidelines carefully.

Herbal Topical

Herbal Balms and Salves: Topical applications of herbs are great for skin issues. Infuse herbs into carrier oils like coconut or olive oil and create balms that can be applied externally.

Usage: Gently massage the herbal balm onto the affected area, ensuring it's safe for your dog's skin.

Seek Professional Advice

While creating herbal preparations can be rewarding, it's essential to consult with a veterinarian or herbalist before introducing new herbs or treatments to your dog. Professional guidance ensures you're using the right herbs, dosages, and methods for your dog's specific needs.

Tailored and Thoughtful

By mastering the art of creating herbal preparations, you're customizing your dog's care routine to their individual needs. The ability to craft infusions, decoctions, tinctures, and topicals empowers you to provide targeted support that nurtures their well-being.

Remember, the goal is not just to administer herbs, but to integrate them thoughtfully into your dog's lifestyle. Through knowledge, care, and the guidance of professionals, you're making a meaningful contribution to your dog's health and happiness.

Dosage and Safety

While creating herbal preparations is empowering, ensuring your dog's safety is paramount. Dosage guidelines are important, as giving too much of an herb can lead to adverse effects. Always start with a low dose and gradually increase, monitoring your dog's response.

Caution: Some herbs can interact with medications or have toxic effects in high doses. Always consult with a veterinarian before introducing new herbs to your dog's routine.

Quality Measures

The quality of the herbs you use directly affects the potency and safety of your preparations. Opt for organic, pesticide-free herbs from reputable sources. If you're sourcing herbs from your garden, ensure they're free from harmful chemicals.

Creating Herbal Blends

Herbal synergy is a powerful concept. Some herbs work better together, enhancing each other's effects. Experimenting with herbal blends allows you to address multiple aspects of your dog's health at once.

Usage: When creating blends, consider consulting with a veterinarian or herbalist to ensure compatibility and appropriate ratios.

Record Keeping

Keeping a journal of your dog's herbal journey can be invaluable. Note the herbs you've used, dosages, and their effects. This record will help you track your dog's progress and adjust your approach over time.

Integrating into Daily Life

Incorporating herbal preparations seamlessly into your dog's daily routine enhances their effectiveness. Whether it's a morning herbal infusion, a soothing balm application, or a tincture added to meals, consistency is key.

Holistic Wellness

While herbal remedies offer significant benefits, they are just one aspect of your dog's overall wellness. Proper nutrition, regular exercise, mental stimulation, and regular veterinary care create a holistic approach to their health.

By mastering the art of creating herbal preparations, you're becoming a proactive advocate for your dog's health. Through knowledge, care, and ongoing learning, you're nurturing your dog's vitality and longevity in a way that aligns with nature's gifts.

CHAPTER 9

CONSULTING WITH A VET

Embarking on the journey of using herbal remedies for your dog's health is an exciting endeavor, but it's essential to remember that professional guidance is crucial. In this chapter, we'll delve into the importance of consulting with a veterinarian when integrating herbal preparations into your dog's care routine.

The Role of a Veterinarian

A veterinarian plays a vital role in your dog's overall health and well-being. When it comes to herbal remedies, their expertise is invaluable in ensuring that your dog receives safe and effective treatment. A veterinarian can provide personalized advice based on your dog's medical history, current health status, and specific needs.

Customized Recommendations

Every dog is unique, and what works well for one dog might not be suitable for another. A veterinarian experienced in herbal medicine can tailor recommendations to your dog's individual characteristics. They can guide you in selecting the right herbs, determining appropriate dosages, and addressing any potential interactions with existing health conditions or medications.

Herbal Safety

One of the most critical aspects of using herbal remedies is ensuring your dog's safety. Certain herbs can have contraindications with medical conditions or medications your dog may be on. A veterinarian can help identify potential risks and advise on the safe use of herbs.

Monitoring and Adjustment

A veterinarian can monitor your dog's progress as you integrate herbal preparations into their routine. Regular check-ins and evaluations help track your dog's response to the herbs and allow for adjustments to be made if necessary. If you're not seeing the desired effects or if there are unexpected changes, a veterinarian can guide you in modifying your approach.

Professional Collaboration

Collaborating with a veterinarian creates a holistic and comprehensive approach to your dog's health. Integrating herbal remedies into your dog's care routine alongside professional veterinary guidance ensures that your dog's well-being is the top priority.

Empowered and Informed

By consulting with a veterinarian, you're arming yourself with the knowledge and guidance needed to make informed decisions about your dog's health. Their expertise and partnership empower you to provide the best care possible for your furry companion.

As you navigate the world of herbal preparations, remember that a veterinarian is an essential member of your dog's healthcare team. With their support, you can confidently harness the benefits of herbs while safeguarding your dog's health and happiness.

Finding a Veterinarian

When seeking a veterinarian's guidance for integrating herbal preparations, it's important to find a professional who is knowledgeable and experienced in both conventional veterinary medicine and herbal remedies. Look for veterinarians who have a background in holistic or integrative medicine, as they are likely to have a deeper understanding of herbal treatments.

Initial Consultation

During the initial consultation, your veterinarian will gather information about your dog's medical history, current health status, and any ongoing treatments or medications. Be prepared to discuss your goals for using herbal remedies and any specific concerns you have about your dog's health.

Tailored Recommendations

Based on the information you provide, your veterinarian will offer tailored recommendations for herbal preparations that align with your dog's needs. They will guide you in selecting the right herbs, determining appropriate dosages, and advising on the best methods of administration.

Monitoring Progress

Your veterinarian will play a crucial role in monitoring your dog's progress as you integrate herbal preparations into their routine. They may schedule follow-up appointments to assess your dog's response, make any necessary adjustments, and address any questions or concerns you may have.

Addressing Concerns

If you have any concerns about your dog's response to herbal remedies, potential side effects, or interactions with medications, your veterinarian is the best person to consult. They can provide accurate information and guide you in making informed decisions about your dog's care.

A Holistic Approach

Working collaboratively with a veterinarian offers a holistic approach to your dog's health. By combining the knowledge of traditional veterinary medicine with the benefits of herbal remedies, you're providing your dog with a comprehensive and well-rounded healthcare plan.

Empowering Your Role

Consulting with a veterinarian empowers you to take a proactive and informed role in your dog's health. You'll gain confidence in your ability to provide the best care possible while benefiting from the expertise of a trained professional.

As you integrate herbal preparations into your dog's care routine, remember that your veterinarian is your ally in this journey. Their guidance ensures that you're using herbs safely and effectively, enhancing your dog's well-being and quality of life.

CONCLUSION

As you reach the end of this journey through the world of herbal remedies for your dog's health, you've embarked on a path that blends tradition, nature, and modern knowledge. By exploring the benefits of various herbs and learning how to create effective preparations, you've gained the tools to enhance your dog's well-being in a holistic and natural way.

Throughout this book, we've touched on the importance of consulting with a veterinarian, tailoring herbal remedies to your dog's needs, and integrating them into a comprehensive care routine. By seeking professional guidance, you've shown your dedication to your dog's health and happiness.

Remember that each dog is unique, and their response to herbal remedies may vary. It's crucial to start slowly, observe your dog's reactions, and make adjustments as needed. The partnership between you, your veterinarian, and the power of nature's remedies will guide you in providing the best possible care for your beloved canine companion.

As you continue on this journey, may the knowledge you've gained empower you to foster your dog's vitality, comfort, and longevity. With the wisdom of herbal remedies and the love you share, you're creating a brighter, healthier future for your furry friend.

Embracing a Natural Connection

By embracing herbal remedies for your dog's health, you're not just tapping into the healing potential of nature; you're deepening the bond you share with your canine companion. Your efforts to provide comfort, support, and well-being reflect the care and love you have for your dog.

A Lifelong Learning Journey

The world of herbs is vast and ever-evolving. As you continue on this journey, consider it a lifelong learning experience. Keep exploring new herbs, refining your herbal preparations, and staying informed about the latest research and developments in herbal medicine for dogs.

Spreading the Knowledge

As you become more proficient in using herbal remedies for your dog, consider sharing your knowledge with fellow dog owners. Your insights and experiences can inspire others to explore natural ways of caring for their pets, creating a positive ripple effect within the canine community.

Gratitude and Fulfillment

At the heart of using herbal remedies for your dog's health is a sense of gratitude for the gift of companionship they bring into your life. Your dedication to their well-being is a testament to the special bond you share, and the moments of joy, comfort, and fulfillment are your reward.

A Healthier Future

By embracing the power of herbs, you're contributing to a healthier future for your dog. Whether it's supporting their immune system, soothing their anxiety, or enhancing their joint mobility, you're enabling them to lead a happier and more vibrant life.

The Lasting Legacy

As you close the chapter on this book, remember that the knowledge you've gained and the love you've shared with your dog will create a lasting legacy. Your commitment to their health and happiness will leave an indelible mark on their journey and the memories you've crafted together.

With herbal remedies, you're not just addressing physical needs; you're nurturing their emotional well-being, and enriching their life in ways that only a caring guardian can. May this journey continue to inspire and guide you on the path of holistic and compassionate care for your cherished canine companion.

www.ingramcontent.com/pod-product-compliance
Lightning Source LLC
Chambersburg PA
CBHW062342290526
45794CB00005B/2080